THE SCIENCE BEHIND HEALTHY LIVING AND FITNESS

HOW EXERCISE IMPACTS THE BODY AND MIND

VICTOR OBIOSA

ISBN: 9798391666769

DEDICATION

This book is dedicated to everyone living an unhealthy lifestyle.

CONTENTS

1 Introduction

2 Understanding the Body

3 Exercise Physiology

4 The Mind-Body Connection

5 Exercise and Specific Populations

6 Lifestyle Factors

7 Overcoming Barriers

8 Conclusion

INTRODUCTION

Welcome to "The Science Behind Healthy Living and Fitness, Including How Exercise Impacts the Body and Mind." In today's world, our lives have become increasingly busy and stressful, leaving little time for self-care and healthy living. However, it is essential to prioritize our health and well-being if we want to lead fulfilling and productive lives. This is where the importance of healthy living and fitness comes in. Healthy living and fitness are not just about looking good or losing weight; they are about taking care of our bodies and minds. They help us reduce the risk of chronic diseases, improve our mental health, and increase our longevity.

This book aims to provide a comprehensive understanding of the science behind healthy living and fitness. It covers the essential components of healthy living, including nutrition, exercise physiology, the mind-body connection, lifestyle factors, and overcoming barriers. Through this book, you will learn about the different types of exercise and their benefits, how the body processes food, the role of hormones in exercise, and how exercise impacts mental health and stress reduction. You will also explore fitness for specific populations such as seniors, children, adolescents, pregnant women, and individuals with chronic health conditions.

Additionally, this book covers the importance of sleep, social support, and reducing sedentary behaviour in healthy living. You will also learn about setting achievable goals and the role of self-compassion in maintaining healthy habits. By the end of this book, you will have a solid understanding of the science behind healthy living and fitness, and how to make sustainable lifestyle changes to optimize your health and well-being. Whether you are a beginner or an experienced fitness enthusiast, this book will equip you with the knowledge and tools you need to prioritize your physical and mental health.

UNDERSTANDING THE BODY

Our bodies are incredibly complex machines, and understanding how they function is essential to achieving optimal health and fitness. In this chapter, we will explore the role of nutrition in overall health, how the body processes food, the importance of micronutrients, and the dangers of processed food and sugar.

The Role of Nutrition in Overall Health

Nutrition plays a crucial role in overall health and well-being. The food we eat provides the building blocks for our bodies to function properly. A diet that is high in nutrients can help prevent chronic diseases, such as heart disease, diabetes, and cancer. It is important to consume a balanced diet that includes a variety of whole foods, such as fruits, vegetables, lean proteins, and whole grains.

How the body processes food

The process of digestion begins in the mouth, where food is broken down by enzymes in our saliva. From there, food travels through the oesophagus and into the stomach, where it is further broken down by stomach acid. The small intestine then absorbs nutrients from the food, which are transported to the liver for processing. The liver plays a crucial role in regulating the body's metabolism, storing excess nutrients, and breaking down toxins.

The Importance of Micronutrients

Micronutrients, such as vitamins and minerals, are essential for maintaining proper bodily function. They play important roles in everything from energy metabolism to immune function. It is important to consume a variety of micronutrients in adequate amounts to support overall health. Nutrient-dense foods such as leafy greens, nuts, and legumes are excellent sources of micronutrients.

The Dangers of Processed Food and Sugar

Processed foods and added sugars can have detrimental effects on our health. They are often high in calories, sugar, and unhealthy fats, and low in essential nutrients. Overconsumption of processed foods and added sugars has been linked to increased risk of obesity, type 2 diabetes, heart disease, and other chronic conditions. It is important to limit our intake of these foods and focus on consuming whole, nutrient-dense foods. In conclusion, understanding how the body processes food and the importance of proper nutrition is crucial to achieving optimal health and fitness. A balanced diet that includes a variety of whole foods and adequate amounts of micronutrients is essential. Limiting consumption of processed foods and added sugars is also important for reducing the risk of chronic diseases.

EXERCISE PHYSIOLOGY

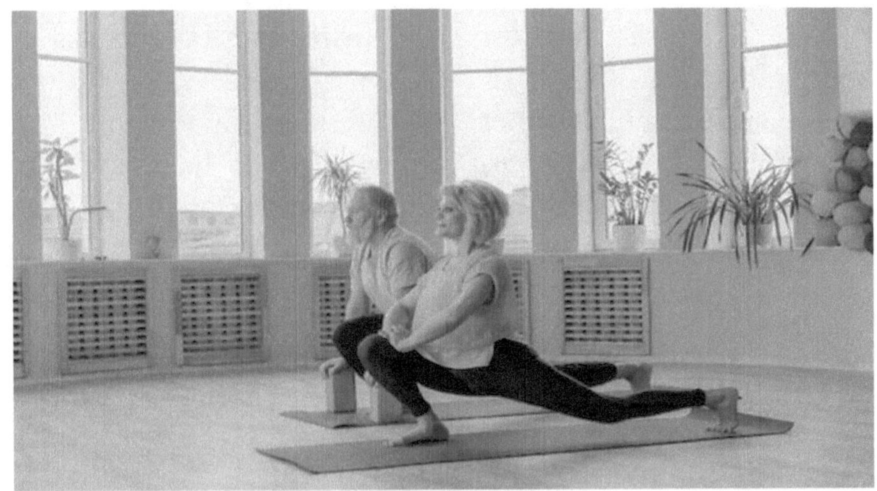

Exercise is a powerful tool for improving overall health and fitness. In this chapter, we will explore different types of exercise and their benefits, the importance of cardiovascular fitness, the role of strength training, understanding the body's response to exercise, and the role of hormones in exercise.

Overview of Different Types of Exercise and Their Benefits

There are various types of exercise that provide different benefits to the body. Aerobic exercise, such as running and cycling, improves cardiovascular health, increases endurance, and burns calories. Resistance training, such as weight lifting, builds muscle mass, increases strength, and improves bone density. Flexibility and balance exercises, such as yoga and Pilates, improve flexibility and balance, which can reduce the risk of falls and injury.

The Importance of Cardiovascular Fitness

Cardiovascular fitness is essential for overall health. Regular aerobic exercise strengthens the heart and lungs, improves circulation, and reduces the risk of cardiovascular disease. It also increases endurance, which can improve overall energy levels and help individuals perform daily activities with greater ease.

The Role of Strength Training

Strength training is important for building muscle mass and increasing strength. This type of exercise can improve bone density, reduce the risk of injury, and enhance overall physical performance. Additionally, increased muscle mass can boost metabolism and help individuals burn more calories even when at rest.

Understanding the Body's Response to Exercise

When we exercise, our bodies undergo various physiological changes. The heart rate increases to pump more blood and oxygen to the working muscles, and the lungs work harder to provide the body with more oxygen. The muscles use stored energy, such as glycogen, and produce waste products, such as lactic acid. Over time, these physiological changes result in improved cardiovascular and muscular endurance.

The Role of Hormones in Exercise

Exercise has a profound impact on hormone levels in the body. For example, exercise can stimulate the release of endorphins, which can improve mood and reduce feelings of stress and anxiety. Exercise can also increase levels of growth hormone, which plays a key role in muscle growth and repair. Other hormones, such as cortisol and insulin, can also be affected by exercise, and can impact overall health and fitness.

In conclusion, understanding exercise physiology is essential for achieving optimal health and fitness. Incorporating different types of exercise, such as aerobic exercise, resistance training, and flexibility and balance exercises, can provide a range of benefits to the body. Cardiovascular fitness and strength training are particularly important for improving overall health, and understanding the body's response to exercise and the role of hormones can help individuals maximize the benefits of their workouts

THE MIND-BODY MECHANISM

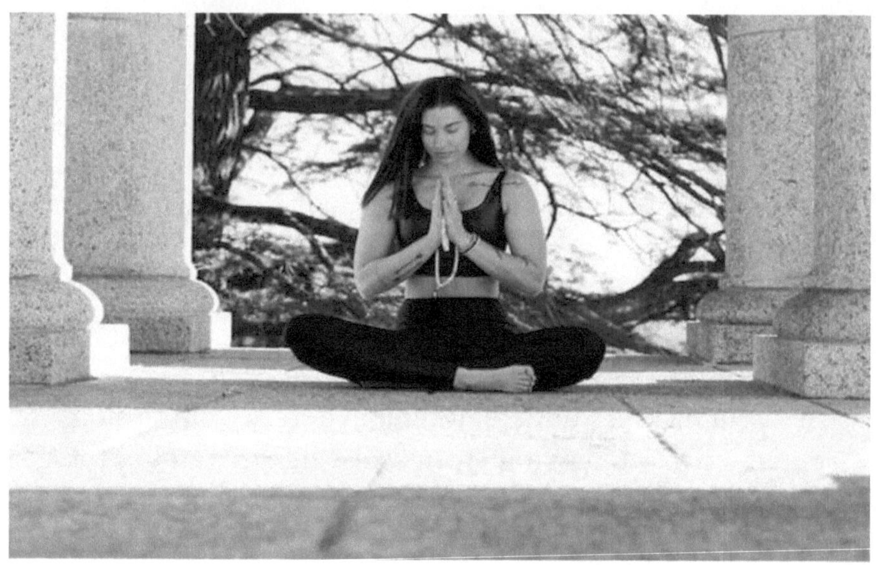

The mind and body are inextricably linked, and understanding this connection is crucial for achieving optimal health and wellness. In this chapter, we will explore how exercise impacts mental health, the relationship between exercise and stress reduction, how exercise can improve mood and cognitive function, and the role of mindfulness and meditation.

How Exercise Impacts Mental Health

Exercise has numerous benefits for mental health, including reducing symptoms of anxiety and depression, improving mood, and enhancing overall well-being. Regular exercise has been shown to increase the production of endorphins, which are the body's natural "feel-good" chemicals. Exercise can also improve self-esteem and reduce social withdrawal and isolation.

The Relationship between Exercise and Stress Reduction

Stress is a common experience for many people, and it can have a significant impact on physical and mental health. Exercise is a powerful tool for reducing stress and managing its negative effects. Exercise can help to regulate stress hormones like cortisol and adrenaline, and it can promote relaxation and a sense of calm.

How Exercise Can Improve Mood and Cognitive Function

Exercise has been shown to improve mood and cognitive function in a number of ways. Regular exercise can enhance cognitive function and improve memory and attention. Exercise can also promote the growth of new brain cells and help to protect existing brain cells from damage.

The Role of Mindfulness and Meditation

Mindfulness and meditation are powerful tools for improving mental health and well-being. Mindfulness involves paying attention to the present moment in a non-judgmental way, while meditation involves focusing the mind on a particular object or thought. Both mindfulness and meditation have been shown to reduce symptoms of anxiety and depression, improve mood, and enhance overall well-being.

In conclusion, understanding the mind-body connection is essential for achieving optimal health and wellness. Exercise has numerous benefits for mental health, including reducing symptoms of anxiety and depression, improving mood and cognitive function, and promoting relaxation and a sense of calm. Mindfulness and meditation are also powerful tools for improving mental health and well-being, and they can be incorporated into a regular exercise routine to enhance its benefits.

EXERCISE AND SPECIFIC POPULATIONS

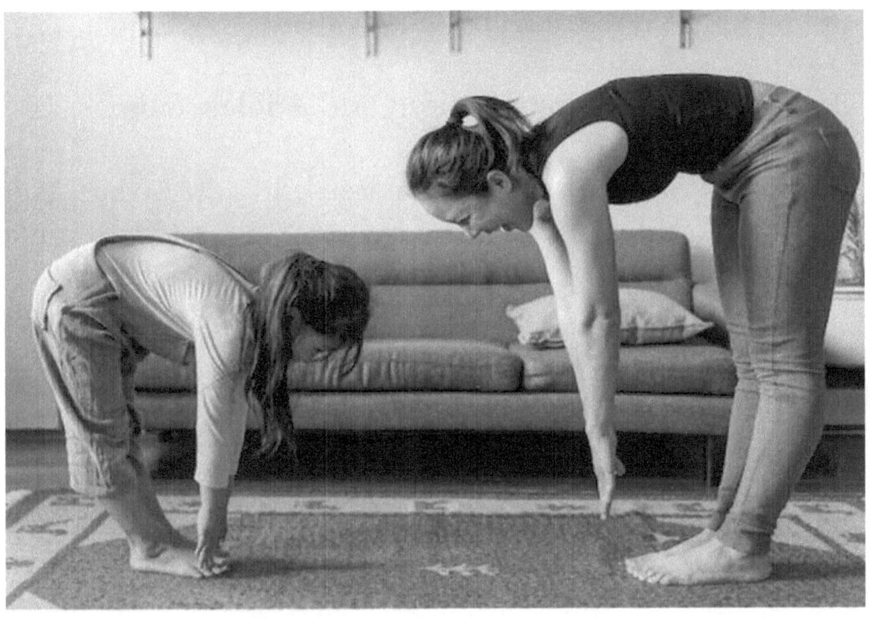

Exercise is crucial for people of all ages and abilities. However, it's important to note that different populations may have different exercise needs and limitations. In this chapter, we will explore the importance of exercise for specific populations, including seniors, children and adolescents, pregnant women, and individuals with chronic health conditions.

Fitness for Seniors

As we age, our bodies undergo changes that can make it harder to maintain overall health and fitness. Exercise can help seniors maintain strength, balance, and mobility, reducing the risk of falls and other injuries. Low-impact exercises like walking, swimming, and yoga can be beneficial for seniors, as well as strength training exercises that focus on building and maintaining muscle mass.

Fitness for Children and Adolescents

Exercise is important for children and adolescents as it promotes healthy growth and development. Children should be encouraged to engage in physical activities they enjoy, such as playing sports, dancing, or playing outside. It's recommended that children and adolescents get at least one hour of physical activity per day.

Fitness for Pregnant Women

Pregnancy can present unique challenges when it comes to exercise, but staying active during pregnancy can have numerous benefits for both the mother and the baby. Exercise during pregnancy can help manage weight gain, reduce the risk of gestational diabetes and high blood pressure, and improve mood and sleep. Low-impact exercises like walking, swimming, and prenatal yoga can be beneficial for pregnant women, but it's important to consult with a healthcare provider before starting any new exercise program.

Fitness for Individuals with Chronic Health Conditions

Exercise can be an important part of managing chronic health conditions such as diabetes, heart disease, and arthritis. In many cases, exercise can help improve symptoms and overall quality of life. However, it's important to work with a healthcare provider to develop an exercise program that is safe and appropriate for the individual's specific condition and needs.

In this chapter, we have explored the importance of exercise for specific populations, including seniors, children and adolescents, pregnant women, and individuals with chronic health conditions. By understanding the unique exercise needs and limitations of these populations, we can develop exercise programs that are safe, effective, and enjoyable for all.

LIFESTYLE FACTORS

Living a healthy and fit lifestyle is not just about exercise and nutrition, but also about other lifestyle factors that can impact overall health and well-being. This chapter will focus on three key factors: sleep, social support, and sedentary behaviour. How Sleep Impacts Overall Health Sleep is essential for overall health and well-being. Getting enough sleep is important for physical, mental, and emotional health. Lack of sleep can contribute to a variety of health issues, such as weight gain, depression, and weakened immune system. In this section, we will discuss the importance of sleep and provide tips for improving sleep quality.

The Role of Social Support in Healthy Living

Social support is crucial for maintaining a healthy lifestyle. It can come from family, friends, or a community. Having a supportive network can help individuals stay motivated, accountable, and encouraged to reach their fitness and health goals. In this section, we will discuss the importance of social support and provide tips for finding and building a supportive network. The

Importance of Reducing Sedentary Behaviour

In today's world, many people spend a large portion of their day sitting or engaging in sedentary behaviour, such as watching TV or sitting at a desk. This can have negative impacts on overall health and well-being, regardless of how much exercise a person does. In this section, we will discuss

the importance of reducing sedentary behaviour and provide
tips for increasing physical activity throughout the day.

OVERCOMING BARRIERS

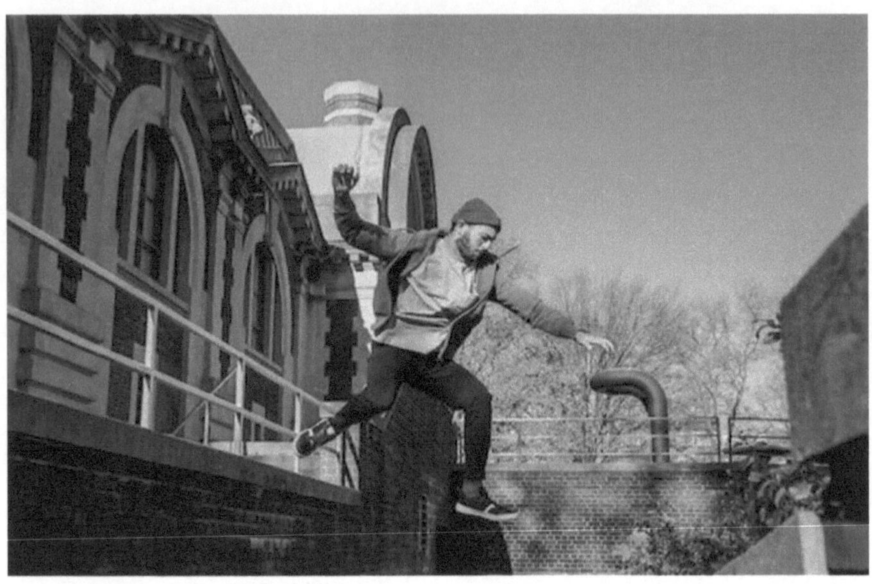

Living a healthy lifestyle and incorporating fitness into our daily routines can be challenging. In this chapter, we'll discuss some common barriers to healthy living and fitness and provide strategies for overcoming them.

Addressing Common Barriers to Healthy Living and Fitness

Some common barriers to healthy living and fitness include lack of time, motivation, knowledge, and access to resources. It's important to recognize and acknowledge these barriers, but it's equally important to find ways to overcome them.

One strategy is to prioritize your health by scheduling exercise into your day and planning healthy meals ahead of time. You can also seek out support from family, friends, or a fitness community to help you stay motivated and accountable.

How to Set Achievable Goals

Setting achievable goals is essential for success in fitness and healthy living. When setting goals, it's important to make them specific, measurable, attainable, relevant, and time-bound (SMART). This helps you stay focused and motivated, and allows you to track your progress. For example, instead of setting a general goal of "losing weight," make it more specific by setting a goal to lose a certain amount of weight in a specific timeframe. This makes the goal more measurable and attainable.

The Role of Self-Compassion in Maintaining Healthy Habits

Self-compassion is an important component of maintaining healthy habits. It involves treating yourself with kindness, understanding, and forgiveness when you face setbacks or challenges. This allows you to be more resilient and motivated to continue working toward your goals. Instead of being overly critical of yourself when you miss a workout or indulge in an unhealthy meal, practice self-compassion by recognizing that setbacks are a normal part of the process and that you can always get back on track.

In conclusion, by addressing common barriers, setting achievable goals, and practicing self-compassion, you can overcome obstacles and maintain a healthy lifestyle. Remember that small, consistent steps can lead to big changes over time.

CONCLUSION

Congratulations! You have reached the end of "The Science Behind Healthy Living and Fitness, Including How Exercise Impacts the Body and Mind." Throughout this book, we have explored the many ways in which exercise and healthy living can impact your body and mind.

Here are some of the key takeaways

1. Healthy living and regular exercise are essential for overall health and well-being.
2. Nutrition plays a critical role in maintaining good health, and we should aim to consume a balanced diet that includes plenty of whole foods and micronutrients.
3. Different types of exercise have unique benefits, but both cardiovascular and strength training exercises are important for overall fitness.
4. Exercise can improve mental health, reduce stress, and improve cognitive function.
5. Specific populations, including seniors, children and adolescents, pregnant women, and those with chronic health conditions, should engage in appropriate exercise for their unique needs.
6. Adequate sleep, social support, and reducing sedentary behavior are all important lifestyle factors that can impact our health.
7. Common barriers to healthy living and fitness can be addressed through goal-setting and self-compassion.

Remember, living a healthy lifestyle is a journey, not a destination. It's essential to take small steps every day to improve your health and well-being. We hope that this book has inspired you to take action and make positive changes in your life.

Thank you for reading "The Science Behind Healthy Living and Fitness, Including How Exercise Impacts the Body and Mind." Best of luck on your journey towards a healthier and happier life!

ABOUT THE AUTHOR

Victor Obiosa is a skilled and experienced writer with a passion for creating engaging and informative articles. He has a natural talent for crafting content that captivates readers and keeps them engaged from beginning to end. Victor has demonstrated his ability to write on a wide variety of topics, including technology, health, lifestyle, business, and finance, among others.